DIETRY FAT IS GREAT FOR WOMEN MENOPAUSE

By

CYNTHIA L. JONES

TABLE OF CONTENTS

TITLE PAGE
TABLE OF CONTENTS
COPYRIGHT ©
INTRODUCTION:
What is menopause
PART I
Is Menopause Good?
PART II
Treatment for Menopause
PART III
Your Diet and Menopause
PART IV
Body Balance: a resultant effect
of fat

INTRODUCTION
What is menopause?

A woman has entered the menopausal stage of life when her menstrual periods end permanently. This stage—often referred to as the "transition of life"—marks the cessation of a woman's potential to become a mother. The time when a woman's hormone levels start to change is often referred to as the menopause by healthcare professionals. Menstrual periods must stop for a full year in order for menopause to be considered complete.

Premenopause is a common name for the time just before menopause. The amount of mature eggs in a woman's ovaries decreases during this transitional period prior to menopause, and ovulation becomes erratic. Progesterone and estrogen production both fall at the same time. It's the significant decline in estrogen that causes most of the signs of menopause in women.

When does menopause begin?

Menopause can happen at any time between the thirties and the mid-fifties, although it typically happens about age 51. Menopause often occurs earlier in smokers and underweight women than in overweight women. Usually, a woman goes through menopause at the same time her mother did.

Menopause can happen for additional reasons besides those that are naturally occurring. These include:

- **_Premature menopause_**
  Premature menopause could come from ovarian failure that happens before the age of 40. It may be caused by smoking, radiation exposure, chemotherapy drugs, or ovarian blood supply-affecting surgery. This is also known as ovarian insufficiency.
- **_Menopause after surgery._**
  Following the removal of one or both ovaries, or the radiation of the pelvis, which includes the ovaries, in premenopausal

women, surgical menopause may occur. This causes a hasty menopause. Compared to women who experience menopause naturally, these women frequently experience more severe menopausal symptoms. Succinctly, As a woman's menstrual cycles come to an end, menopause is a normal life transition. Hormone fluctuations can result in symptoms like night sweats and poor sleep and may have a negative impact on metabolism and bone density.

Your endocrine system (Your Hormones Production)

You need as many hormones as you can obtain during the peri-menopause and the menopause. And in order to generate hormones, we need to consume a particular amount of fat in our diet.

Looking at a lot of study over the past few years, I discovered something extremely intriguing: those of you who are currently going through the peri-menopause and the menopause are the women who were raised being told that obesity is evil and the enemy. Being on a low-fat diet for almost your entire life as you approach menopause and the peri-menopause may be having an effect on your hormonal health at this time

Dietary fats are necessary to fuel your body and maintain cell function. They also aid in keeping your body warm and in defending your organs. Your body utilizes fats to release pivotal hormones and to absorb certain nutrients. As you read on, you'll discover how body fat (dietry fat) which has been labelled has "evil" has a lot of positive contribution to add to your menopausal experience.

PART I
Is Menopause Good?

Like many women, you might be a little startled to learn that menopause can improve your life. Hot flashes, vaginal dryness, mood swings, receding hair, and sleep difficulties are just a few of the unpleasant symptoms that come to mind when thinking of menopause. It's a long and depressing list. Though not all bodily changes brought on by lower levels of female hormones are bad, menopause can nevertheless have a positive effect on your life. Another reason is that a lot of the psychological and social changes can actually be stimulating. Discover what many women have already learned by reading on: Menopause can bring about a lot of positive changes. These changes includes:

No more (Premenstrual syndrome) PMS

Premenstrual syndrome (PMS) can result in a wide range of physical and mental symptoms, from breast soreness and headache pain to food cravings and irritability, in the week or two prior to your period. According to the American College of Obstetricians and Gynecologists, at least 85% of all women who are menstruating suffer one or more PMS symptoms each month. As estrogen levels fluctuate during the perimenopause, PMS may briefly get worse. So it's much better if PMS goes away after menopause. There is no doubt that menopause can be a "Ahhhh!" kind of period for women, most especially for those who have experienced mood changes akin to these hormonal fluxes, according to Dr. Stuenkel. "Perimenopause involves some years of a very rough hormonal variance," she adds.

Sex without pregnancy worries

Menopausal women can have intercourse without worrying about getting pregnant. The Investigation of Women's Health Across the Nation, a multisite, longitudinal study of the physical and psychosocial changes women encounter in midlife, including menopause, finds that this has a significant impact. One advantage of menopause, according to Nanette Santoro, MD, professor and director of Reproductive Endocrinology at Albert Einstein College of Medicine in New York, is the ability to have sex without worrying about getting pregnant. Some women even discover that as they enter menopause, they are able to enjoy sex more since they are no longer concerned about its unexpected results

The end of Hormonal Headache

According to the National Headache Foundation, women get headaches three times more frequently than men do. Menstrual migraines, headaches that occur at the same time as ovulation and menstruation, affect about 70% of these women. These headaches, like other migraines, are characterized by throbbing pain on one side of the head, which is occasionally followed by nausea, vomiting, and sensitivity to light or sound. Variations in estrogen and progesterone levels during a regular menstrual cycle might result in menstrual migraines. However, estrogen and progesterone levels drop after menopause, and frequently, so do the frequency of hormonal headaches. Dr. Santoro says that migraine sufferers can anticipate relief once they have passed the menopause transition. "Headaches can temporarily worsen during the turbulent hormone changes associated with perimenopause," she says.

Naturally, uterine fibroids decrease

Fibroids are uterine tumors that commonly affect women who are close to menopause and are virtually always benign. During pregnancy, when progesterone and estrogen levels rise, and in perimenopause, when estrogen levels can fluctuate from low to high, fibroids develop when the body's estrogen levels are high. Doctors may advise surgery if fibroid symptoms, including as pain, heavy menstrual blood, and pressure on the bladder, are severe. Fortunately, when women hit menopause and their estrogen levels drop, fibroids frequently stop growing or even shrink. Menopause is beneficial for women who have been tracking fibroid growth in an effort to prevent surgery or for those whose heavy periods are brought on by fibroids. Menopause gives women who have fibroids pressing against their bladder a break!

Greater self assurance

Because of the physiologic changes that occur during menopause as well as the stage of life at which menopause occurs, it's not unusual for postmenopausal women to report being empowered. Women frequently express relief at not experiencing monthly periods and the associated risk of pregnancy, mood swings, and other PMS symptoms, according to Dr. Richardson. "At the same time, as your kids become older, you have more time to pursue your career and personal goals." Women are more likely to go for what they want with a greater sense of confidence that they can handle anything that comes their way after 50+ years of life experience, including the ups and downs of marriages, childrearing, and professions.

A chance to take stock

The surge of energy that some women experience after menopause is known as "menopausal zest" by American anthropologist Margaret Mead. As a result, women naturally reflect on their lives during menopause. Many people make the decision to reevaluate their relationships, careers, methods of self-care, and preferred outlets for their energy. Dr. Stuenkel emphasizes the significance of seizing this opportunity to say, "Let's put our best foot forward as we move along." She counsels menopausal women to assess their progress in both their professional and personal lives, as well as whether the way they are spending their time is meaningful to them.

A time to take a chance

According to Dr. Stuenkel, "we used to say you are left with a third of your life after menopause." "Now, however, I advise ladies that they only have half a life left. The party has begun; stop being reserved." Women going through menopause are particularly in need of hearing this message because midlife is a time when they are more likely to take risks. Some people change occupations, possibly expanding a pastime into a business. Others try figure skating, internet dating, or other risk-taking activities like mountain climbing. There is no better moment than the present to experience all life has to offer, if there is something you've been putting off

Focus on caring for yourself

Women in menopause have more time to take care of themselves because their children are grown or on their way to independence and have established careers. " There has never been a better time to overhaul your health. Many women going through menopause are open to making changes that will keep or improve their health. These adjustments can begin with routine health screenings and checkups. You can also put your best foot forward by following a healthy diet that's low in fat and high in fruits and vegetables, as well as by engaging in regular physical activity — by walking and biking to gardening down to doing house chore counts. Finally, it's crucial to decompress and lessen stress; tai chi, relaxation exercises, and meditation are some of the tools that can do this.

Bonding with other menopausal women

You may identify with any woman who is as sweaty or forgetful as yourself when heat flashes have you removing layers of clothing or when you can't remember what it was you came to the store for. By letting you know that you're not alone, talking — and frequently laughing — with other women about the menopausal symptoms you're going through can be quite beneficial. In addition to exchanging coping mechanisms, sympathies, and understanding, Dr. Richardson claims that women who share their tales gain strength from knowing that they are not alone and that unwanted symptoms will pass.

PART II
Treatment for menopause

No medical care is necessary during menopause. Instead, treatments concentrate on controlling or avoiding chronic illnesses that may develop with aging as well as curing your indications and symptoms. Treatments could consist of:

Hormone therapy: The most effective method of treating menopausal heat flashes is estrogen medication. Your doctor may advise estrogen in the lowest dose and shortest time period necessary to relieve your symptoms, depending on your personal and family medical history. You will require progestin in addition to estrogen if your uterus is still present. Estrogen also helps stop bone thinning. Although initiating hormone therapy around menopause has proven benefits for some women, long-term usage of hormone therapy may carry some cardiovascular and breast cancer concerns. Speak to your physician about the benefits and risks of hormone therapy and if it's a safe option for you.

Vaginal lotion: Using a vaginal lotion, pill, or ring, estrogen can be directly delivered to the vagina to treat vaginal dryness. Only a tiny amount of estrogen is released during this procedure, and it is absorbed by the vaginal tissues. Vaginal dryness, discomfort during sexual activity, and some urinary symptoms can all be helped by it.

Low-dose antidepressants: SSRIs, a type of antidepressants that includes certain antidepressants (Selective Serotonin Reuptake inhibitors) are thought to lessen menopausal heat flashes. Women who need an antidepressant for a mood condition or who are unable to take estrogen may find relief from hot flashes with a low-dose antidepressant.

Gabapentin (Gralise, Horizant, Neurontin): Gabapentin has been demonstrated to help lessen hot flashes in addition to being approved to treat seizures. Women who cannot utilize estrogen therapy or who additionally experience overnight hot flashes can benefit from this medication.

Clonidine (Catapres, Kapvay): Hot flashes may be somewhat alleviated by clonidine, a tablet or patch generally used to treat high blood pressure

Drugs that either treat or prevent osteoporosis: Doctors may provide medicine to treat or prevent osteoporosis depending on the needs of the patient. Several drugs are available that help lower the risk of fractures and bone loss. To assist strengthen your bones, your doctor may advise taking vitamin D pills.

Discuss your options and the risks and benefits of each with your doctor before deciding on a course of therapy. Every year, reevaluate your alternatives because your needs and treatment options might change

You may also try out home remedies options like:

Develop your relaxing skills: Menopausal symptoms may be alleviated by methods including progressive muscle relaxation, guided meditation, deep breathing, and timed breathing. Numerous books and online resources are available that demonstrate various relaxation techniques

Decrease vaginal discomfort
Try using a water-based vaginal lubricant (such as Astroglide, K-Y jelly, Sliquid, or others) or a lubricant or moisturizer with silicone as an alternative (Replens, K-Y Liquibeads, Sliquid, others).

If you are sensitive to glycerin, you may want to select a product without it since it might burn or irritate your skin. By engaging in sexual activities, you will be increasing blood flow to the vagina, and also reducing vaginal discomfort.

Get adequate rest

Avoid coffee, which can make it difficult to fall asleep, and excessive alcohol consumption, which can disrupt sleep. Exercise during the day, but not just before going to bed. Before you can get a good night's sleep if hot flashes keep you up, you may need to figure out how to handle them.

Make your pelvic floor stronger
Exercises for the pelvic floor muscles, or "Kegels," can help some types of urine incontinence.

Consume a healthy diet
A variety of fruits, vegetables, and whole grains should be consumed. Limit sweets, oils, and saturated fats. To help you fulfill daily requirements, inquire with your provider if you need calcium or vitamin D supplements.

Avoid smoking

Smoking raises your risk of developing cancer, osteoporosis, heart disease, a stroke, and a number of other illnesses. Additionally, it might intensify hot flashes and hasten the onset of menopause.

PART III
Your Diet and Menopause

As a woman's menstrual cycles come to an end, menopause is a normal life transition. Twelve months following your last period, it is proven. The menopause transition and its symptoms, however, might extend for a number of years.

Although menopause is associated with a number of unpleasant symptoms and raises your risk of contracting particular diseases, your diet may assist ease the transition and lessen symptoms.

What Alterations Take Place During Menopause?

Your regular cyclical patterns of estrogen and progesterone are disturbed as you approach menopause and beyond because the hormone estrogen starts to diminish. Your metabolism is significantly impacted by declining estrogen levels, which could result in weight gain. Your cholesterol levels and the way your body digests carbohydrates may also be impacted by these changes. During this transitional stage, a lot of women encounter symptoms including hot flashes and trouble sleeping.

Furthermore, hormonal fluctuations cause a decrease in bone density, which can raise your risk of fractures. Thankfully, altering your diet may help reduce menopause symptoms. There is proof that some foods may help with menopause symptoms like hot flashes, poor sleep, and low bone density.

Diary Foods
Women's risk of fractures may rise as a result of the fall in estrogen levels following menopause.

Calcium, phosphorus, potassium, magnesium, and vitamins D and K are all found in dairy products like milk, yogurt, and cheese and are crucial for maintaining healthy bones.

In a study involving approximately 750 postmenopausal women, those who consumed more dairy and animal protein compared favorably with those who consumed less.

Dairy products may also enhance sleep. According to a review study, menopausal women who ate meals high in the amino acid glycine, which is present in dairy products like milk and cheese, reported getting deeper sleep.

Additionally, some research suggests that dairy consumption lowers the incidence of premature menopause, which starts before age 45.

Women in one study who scored the highest consumption of vitamin D and calcium — which are contained in cheese and fortified milk— had a 17% reduction in the risk of early menopause

Healthy Fats

Menopausal women may benefit from consuming healthy fats like omega-3 fatty acids. Omega-3 supplements lessened the frequency of hot flashes and the intensity of night sweats, according to a review research involving 483 menopausal women.

Only a small number of studies, in another analysis of 8 studies on omega-3 and menopausal symptoms, backed the fatty acid's favorable impact on hot flashes. As a result, the findings were not definitive. Even so, it would be worthwhile to investigate whether boosting your omega-3 consumption lessens menopause-related symptoms. The foods with the highest levels of omega-3 fatty acids are seeds like flax, chia, and hemp, as well as fatty fish like mackerel, salmon, and anchovies

Full Grain

The B vitamins thiamine, niacin, riboflavin, and pantothenic acid are among the many nutrients found in whole grains, along with fiber.

A diet rich in whole grains has been associated with a lower risk of cancer, heart disease, and early mortality.

Researchers conducted a review and discovered that persons who had three or more servings of whole grains daily had a 20–30% decreased risk of developing diabetes and heart disease compared to those who consumed predominantly refined carbohydrates.

In comparison to eating merely 1.3 grams of whole-grain fiber per 2,000 calories, consuming 4.7 grams of whole-grain fiber per day lowered the risk of early death by 17%, according to a study involving more than 11,000 postmenopausal women.

Vegetables and fruits

Fruits and vegetables are a great source of fiber, antioxidants, and vitamins and minerals. American nutrition recommendations advise placing fruits and vegetables on half of your plate because of this.

In a one-year intervention research with more than 17,000 menopausal women, those who consumed more vegetables, fruit, fiber, and soy saw a 19% decrease in hot flashes compared to the control group. The healthier diet and weight loss were said to be the causes of the decline.

For postmenopausal women in particular, cruciferous veggies may be beneficial. In one study, eating broccoli increased levels of an estrogen type that protects against breast cancer while decreasing levels of an estrogen type linked to the disease

Additionally advantageous to menopausal women, dark berries. 25 grams of freeze-dried strawberry powder per day reduced blood pressure in comparison to a control group during the course of an eight-week research with 60 menopausal women. However, more investigation is required.

Another eight-week trial included 91 middle-aged women, and those who took supplements containing 200 mg of grape seed extract daily reported fewer hot flashes, better sleep, and lower rates of depression than those in the control group

Phytoestrogens-containing food

Phytoestrogens are substances found in food that function in your body like weakened estrogens.

Even while there has been some debate about adding them in the diet, recent study indicates they may have health benefits, particularly for menopausal women.

Soybeans, chickpeas, peanuts, flax seeds, barley, grapes, cherries, plums, green and black tea, and many more foods naturally contain phytoestrogens.

Postmenopausal women who took soy isoflavone supplements for at least four weeks had 14% greater estradiol (estrogen) levels than those who took a placebo, according to a study of 21 soy trials. Results, though, were not noteworthy. Another evaluation of 15 trials covering a period of three to twelve months discovered that phytoestrogens including soy, isoflavone supplements, and red clover reduced the frequency of hot flashes in comparison to control groups without causing any harmful side effects

Suitable Protein

The loss of estrogen after menopause is associated with a deterioration in bone density and muscular mass.

This is why menopausal women should consume more protein. According to recommendations, women over 50 should consume 20–25 grams of high-quality protein every meal, or 0.4–0.55

grams of protein per pound (1–1.2 grams per kg) of body weight, daily.

For all persons over the age of 18, the Recommended Dietary Allowance (RDA) for protein in the US is 0.36 grams per pound (0.8 grams per kilogram) of body weight, which is the bare minimum required for health. The range for protein in the recommended macronutrient composition is 10–35% of total daily calories

In a recent study, postmenopausal women who consumed 5 grams of collagen peptides daily had considerably higher bone mineral density compared to those who consumed a placebo powder over the course of a year. The majority of the proteins in your body are collagen. In a large study of over-50-year-old adults, consuming dairy protein was associated with an 8% reduction in the risk of hip fracture, while eating plant protein was associated with a 12% decrease. Eggs, meat, fish, lentils, and dairy products are among the foods high in protein. Protein powders can also be added to smoothies or baked goods

Foods to Exclude

Avoiding some foods may help lessen some of the menopause-related symptoms, including hot flashes, weight gain, and restless sleep.

Added sugar and refined carbohydrates

Hot flashes are more common in menopausal women and have been linked to excessive blood sugar, insulin resistance, and metabolic syndrome.

Blood sugar is known to rise quickly in response to processed diets and added sugars. A food's impact on blood sugar may be more pronounced the more processed it is.

As a result, cutting less on processed meals and added sugars like white bread, crackers, and baked goods may help lessen hot flashes during menopause. According to US guidelines, you should consume no more than 10% of your daily calories from added sugars. This means that if you consume 2,000 calories, less than 200 calories, or 50 grams, should come from added sugars.

Caffeine and alcohol

Caffeine and alcohol have been demonstrated in studies to cause heat flashes in menopausal women. In one study, coffee and alcohol consumption increased the intensity of hot flashes but not their frequency in 196 menopausal women. On the other hand, a another study linked coffee use to a decreased risk of hot flashes. It might be worthwhile to evaluate whether giving up caffeine has an impact on your hot flashes. Consider the fact that many women going through menopause have difficulties sleeping, as well as the fact that alcohol and caffeine are known to disturb sleep. Consider avoiding caffeine or alcohol near bedtime if this applies to you.

Sodium-Rich Foods

Lower bone density has been associated with high salt intake in postmenopausal women. A study including more than 9,500 postmenopausal women found that consuming more than 2 grams of sodium daily increased the likelihood of having low bone mineral density by 28%. The decrease in estrogen that occurs after menopause also raises your chance of having high blood pressure. Taking less salt may assist to reduce this risk. In addition, compared to women who followed a generally healthy diet with no salt limitation, those who followed a moderate-sodium diet reported having higher overall moods in a research involving 95 postmenopausal women

Menopause symptoms may be lessened by avoiding processed carbohydrates, added sugars, alcohol, caffeine, spicy meals, and foods high in sodium.
Reduced bone density, altered metabolism, and an elevated risk of heart disease are all associated with menopause.

In addition, a lot of menopausal women have uncomfortable symptoms including hot flashes and restless nights. Menopause symptoms may be lessened by a whole-foods diet rich in fruits, vegetables, whole grains, high-quality protein, and dairy products. Healthy fats like omega-3 fatty acids from fish and phytoestrogens may also be beneficial. You might also want to cut back on alcohol, caffeine, processed carbs, added sweets, foods high in sodium, and spicy foods. This crucial adjustment in your life might be made easier by these straightforward dietary changes.

PART IV
Body balance; a resultant effect of fat

Adipose tissue has other names including fat (body fat).

My adipose tissue—where is it?

Body fat is a frequent term for adipose tissue. It is located everywhere on the body. It can be found in breast tissue, between muscles, within bone marrow, under the skin (subcutaneous fat), and packed around internal organs (visceral fat). Men typically accumulate more visceral fat, or fat around the internal organs, which causes them to be overweight in the centre of their belly. Buttocks and thighs are where women frequently retain the most subcutaneous fat. The sex hormones generated by males and females are responsible for these disparities.

How does adipose tissue function?

It is now recognized that adipose tissue is a crucial and functional endocrine organ. Adipocytes, often known as fat cells, are well known to be essential for the storage and release of energy throughout the human body. Adipose tissue's role in the endocrine system has only lately come to light. Adipocytes are just one type of cell found in adipose tissue, which also has a large number of other cells that can create hormones in response to signals from the body's other organs. Adipose tissue is crucial for controlling the metabolism of sex hormones, cholesterol, and glucose through the activities of these hormones.

What hormones does fat tissue secrete?

From adipose tissue, a variety of hormones are released, and each of these is in charge of a particular bodily function. These are:

- Aromatase, which is involved in the metabolism of sex hormones
- TNF alpha, IL-6, and leptin, collectively known as "cytokines," are involved in communicating between cells.

- Blood clotting is facilitated by plasminogen activator inhibitor-1.
- The hormone angiotensin regulates blood pressure
- Adiponectin, which increases the body's insulin sensitivity and so aids in preventing type 2 diabetes
- Apolipoprotein E and lipoprotein lipase are enzymes that are involved in the storage and metabolization of fat to provide energy

What may possibly happen to adipose tissue?

Adipose tissue levels that are excessive or too low might have negative effects on health. Obesity is most frequently caused by having too much adipose tissue, particularly visceral fat. Numerous major health issues are brought on by obesity. Because obesity makes the body more resistant to insulin, it raises the risk of type 2 diabetes. High blood sugar levels as a result of this resistance are harmful to health. Additionally, being obese puts one at risk for developing high blood pressure, high cholesterol, and an increased tendency to clot. These all increase the risk of stroke and heart attacks.

What is the most effective strategy to stop weight gain after menopause?

For preventing or reversing menopause weight gain, there is no secret formula. Focus on the basics of weight prevention and management:

Move more

You can lose extra weight and keep it off by engaging in physical activity, such as strength training and aerobic exercise. Gaining muscle helps your body burn calories more effectively, which makes it simpler to maintain a healthy weight. Most healthy individuals should engage in strong aerobic activity, such as jogging, for at least 75 minutes per week, or moderate aerobic activity, such as brisk walking, for at least 150 minutes per week.

Furthermore, weight training exercises should be performed at least twice each week. You might need to exercise more if you want to shed weight or achieve specific fitness goals.

Eat less and eat right

You may require 200 fewer calories per day in your fifties than you needed in your thirties and forties to maintain your weight, much alone shed more pounds. Be mindful of your eating and drinking habits if you want to cut calories without sacrificing nutrition.

Increase your consumption of fruits, vegetables, and whole grains, especially those that are less processed and higher in fiber.

A plant-based diet is often better for you than other options. Good options include fish, soy, almonds, legumes, and low-fat dairy products. Limit your consumption of meat, especially chicken and red meat. Use oils like olive or vegetable oil in place of butter, stick margarine, and shortening.

Inspect your sweet routine

In the typical American diet, added sugars make up roughly 300 calories per day. Most of these calories—about half of them—come from sugar-sweetened liquids such soft drinks, juices, energy drinks, flavored waters, and sweetened coffee and tea. Cookies, pies, cakes, doughnuts, ice cream, and candy are other foods that increase dietary sugar intake.

Alcohol use should be kept to a minimum

Drinking alcohol increases your risk of gaining weight since it adds extra calories to your diet.

Look for help

Be in the company of loved ones and friends who will support your attempts to adopt a healthy diet and improve your level of physical activity. Even better, form a team and alter your lifestyle as a whole.

A lasting change in food and exercise routines is necessary for weight loss success at any stage of life. Dedicate yourself to lifestyle changes and enjoy a healthier you.